COMPULSIVE EATING

How to overcome binge-eating-disorders and re-program your brain to stop being obsessed by hunger. A guide to develop self-confidence by maintaining a mindful and healthy relationship with food.

ADELE ADANI

"There are people in the world so hungry, that God cannot appear to them except in the form of bread."

Mahatma Gandhi.

TABLE OF CONTENT

INTRODUCTION

Compulsive behaviors can be defined as repeated attitudes, despite being inadequate in certain situations. People often recognize that their behavior is harmful, but they feel emotionally compelled to implement it. Compulsion, in general, is linked to obsessive-compulsive disorder, in the non-control of the impulses of substance abuse.

However compulsive behavior is a *modus operandi* not only of substance abuse from addictions, but also of eating disorders, such as the Binge Eating Disorder.

This pathology linked to food is characterized by an immoderate and uncontrollable need to overeat. The control of this behavior is very difficult, despite the attempts undertaken.

The current models to counter the Binge Eating Disorder focus attention on three elements in particular:

1) uncontrolled feeding as a habit;

2) nutrition as a dysfunctional strategy to deal with a negative emotional state;

3) uncontrolled nutrition despite adverse consequences.

Compulsive feeding is characterized by brain dysfunctions in the areas dedicated to learning by reward. The reward system is a group of neural structures responsible for motivation, associative learning and positive emotions, in particular, those that involve pleasure such as, joy, euphoria and ecstasy.

The reward is the motivational property of a stimulus that induces appetitive behavior, also known as consumption behavior, which flows into the Binge Eating Disorder. Understanding how and why this disturbing complex develops is very difficult.

It is good to be wary of those who claim to know what the causes of these ailments are. The reasons are many and probably different from person to person. Although research is becoming increasingly interested in this topic, numerous efforts are still needed to hinder compulsive eating behavior.

Our work aims to improve the prospects of prevention and treatment in a preventive perspective, probing the emotional processes in charge of controlling feelings.

Feelings and emotions live with us, yet many times we pay little attention to our inner experience. We do not see our emotional world as a wealth, a potential. We are more inclined to enhance rational thinking, leaving aside the emotional experience.

In the era in which we find ourselves living, characterized by the desire to posses more, everything immediately in real time, the time for self-reflection is every time less. We live, in fact, in an accelerated world in which everyone is always in a hurry. To understand what is really important it is necessary to stop, re-evaluate ourselves and revisit the emotions experienced. Our experiences accompany us and silently challenge us, call us back, guide us. So it is important to consider emotional dynamisms to better penetrate emotions and evaluate how much they can help us embark on a new lifestyle.

This work is proposed as an attempt to re-evaluate this re-marriage that we have available. The book is divided into six chapters and tries to give useful information for those who, taken by their health problems, seem to ignore every other sphere of humanity and pay attention to feelings and emotions. They therefore grow as emotionally illiterate. They selfishly focus on the relationship of the senses, touch, smell, and of course, above all the taste, which obviously deals with food.

All this must be educated, it must be exercised, it must be formed through constancy and listening to oneself in order to open up to the other. The book will be a training journey to glimpse how, by listening to wisely evaluated advice and indications, it is possible to reach the goal of embarking on a path of authentic socio-affective integration. A part of the book will go into the various ways of countering the Binge Eating Disorder one of the most common ailments in the modern population.

It is a story of the difficult struggle to get out of the disease that affects people and involves their families. Obviously, for a scientific and professional approach to the Binge Eating Disorder, the support of a team of experts is the only solution for the administration of appropriate treatments and therapies to be followed, to effectively tackle the various pathologies. A widely documented reconstruction of all the stages of this long obstacle course has been made, in which food, the body and emotions are the fundamental tools for the rebirth of a new life.

The message is to remember that it is always possible to transform our weak points into an opportunity for growth and gift. Believing that situations of fatigue, anguish, sadness, pain are always in us and give meaning to our life. The realization of the person consisting in continually reaching more, integrated with what he already has, allows you to take a step forward in your existential journey.

1. WE ARE WHAT WE EAT

Philosophy and Food

Eating is universal and the universal, you know, pleases philosophy. However at the same time it has to do with the body, as well as sexuality. Eating goes beyond the biological question and opens up to the dimension of meaning.

Philosophy has always dealt with food, understood both as the primary need of the body and as a metaphor for what nourishes the human. Through the food act, we become what we eat.

The philosophical approach has allowed us to interpret food through a subjective, relational and natural point of view.

Nourishment stimulates our subjective sphere, reassures us and brings us back to the metaphor of the original contact, the maternal one. The analysis of subjectivity within the relationship with food reveals an inevitable relationship with the other. The socio-relational path starts from the maternal body up to the food community to which the individual feels he belongs and which he contributes to determining.

By taking food we assimilate the world is also the comparison with the animal, with whom we share the need for nourishment and consequently the act of eating. Through the alimentary act, we become what we eat. This is a comparison that depresses humans to the bestial condition, flattening them at the level of simple matter. As in other areas, also in relation to food, man is constantly engaged in developing strategies that could definitively indicate a detachment from the animal world.

Medieval thought judges excess food as lust, particularly forms of intemperance of the senses. They are both transgressions of the flesh, respectively, inherent in excess in the food and sexual spheres.

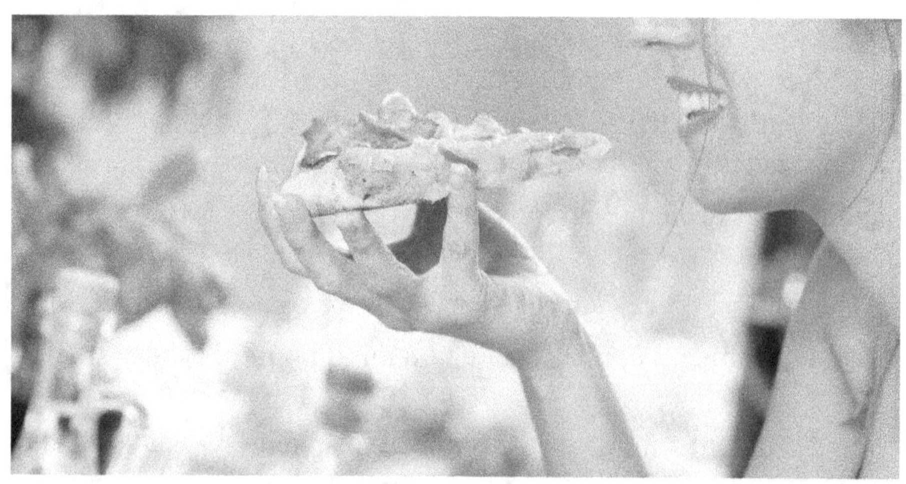

The act of eating is necessarily connected to pleasure. It is difficult to distinguish what is required from necessity and pleasure. Given the physiological need for nourishment, we should be able to discern between need and desire. In the act of eating, we satisfy two types of appetite, the natural appetite, to which belong the primary sensations of hunger and thirst, which refers to need. At the same time, we satisfy the sensory appetite, which presides over the desire for food and tastes.

If we want, this classification allows us to identify the fate of the insatiable from those of the voracious, which sometimes coincides with those affected by the binge eating disorder.

The first has to do with the qualitative refinement of the senses, it does not satisfy itself for the materiality of the food, but for the unbridled exaltation of the sensations of the palate. The second has to do not only with the satisfaction of the physiological need but with the excessive quantity of hunger, therefore, the insatiability of the natural appetite.

Psychology and food

Those affected by binge eating seem to ignore every other sphere of humanity, paying limited attention to the feelings and emotions. Leave out your inner experience, your emotional world. They therefore grow as emotionally illiterate, unrelated to themselves and to what happens inside them, wrapped in a storm of emotions from which they are increasingly dominated and less and less able to learn. Thus we lose contact with that part of us without which it is difficult to lead a peaceful life. He selfishly focuses on the relationship of the senses, the touch, the sense of smell and, of course, above all the taste, which relate it to food. Consequently, the act of eating can be automatic and at the same time full of irreversible consequences, which escape the control and moderation of reason.

The separation between body and reason that has marked philosophy since its inception has meant that philosophy has given only marginal importance to food.

Although once those who ate excessively were opposed, in the eyes of modern sensibility, they no longer seem to be attributable to such a serious lack. Gluttony, from capital transgression, a moral error worthy of eternal punishment has become, for men of the beginning of the third millennium, a venial infringement of the aesthetic order.

To the ethical imperatives of the societies of hunger and shortage, the modern civilization of consumption has replaced the prescriptions, sometimes just as iron and binding for the needs of fashion and the public to appear, of dietetics. They therefore grow as emotionally illiterate, extraneous to themselves and to what happens inside them, wrapped in a storm of emotions from which they are increasingly dominated and less and less able to learn. In the era in which we find ourselves living, characterized by the tendency to want everything immediately in real time, little time is reserved for reflection on oneself. We live, in fact, in an accelerated world in which everyone is always in a hurry, while to understand what is really important it is necessary to stop, re-evaluate, understand with the emotions experienced. Our experiences accompany us, silently challenge us, call us back, guide us. So the intelligence of emotions remains an educational challenge for everyone. Indeed, emotion is not only what happens to us, but above all it is what moves us. So it is important to consider emotional dynamisms. We must not only understand emotions, but evaluate how much these emotions can help us understand.

The message is to remember that it is always possible to transform our weak points into an opportunity for growth and gift, to believe that in situations of fatigue, anguish, sadness pain there is a sense for one's existence, because the realization of the person consists in reaching continuously what more, integrated with what it already has, allows you to take a step forward in our existential journey.

The Consumer Society

In today's obese society there is a perverse combination between the physical feeling of satisfaction and fullness on the one hand and the idea of obeying the norms of insatiable consumption on the other.

To the society of overproduction, much more than bodies that work, they are interested in the bodies that consume. The spirit of capitalism stimulates, the tendency to insatiability and awakens different forms of desire for accumulation.

Everything is mobilized to awaken an ever new hunger, not only for food. An important component of our day is the intake of the products of the media diet. We start from the poorest, consisting only of television and we get to the slightly more moderate one based on TV, radio and newspapers up to the diet rich in new technologies.

Another type of hunger is involved in this area, metaphorically fueled by the connection network, hunger for devices to be consumed, which the appropriate sales centers present, by virtue of shrewd marketing strategies. The sales techniques flatter and pamper the customer, making him feel unique and loved, and present in design packages, true design masterpieces. Therefore both food and electronic gadgets appear to some to be the only thing that can take care of them. For the physiological appetite, the mechanisms are identical. Satisfaction is found in the sweet-soft fat diet, easy and cheap, where the overweight person obediently bends to the ideal of the insatiable consumer who feeds on low-cost foods rich in calories, sugars and fats, salt and yeast.

The mass consumption industry contributes to the spread of food illiteracy and the inability to cook good food, with style and competence, without falling into the trap of the rhetoric of the grandmother's kitchen.

Sedentary lifestyle

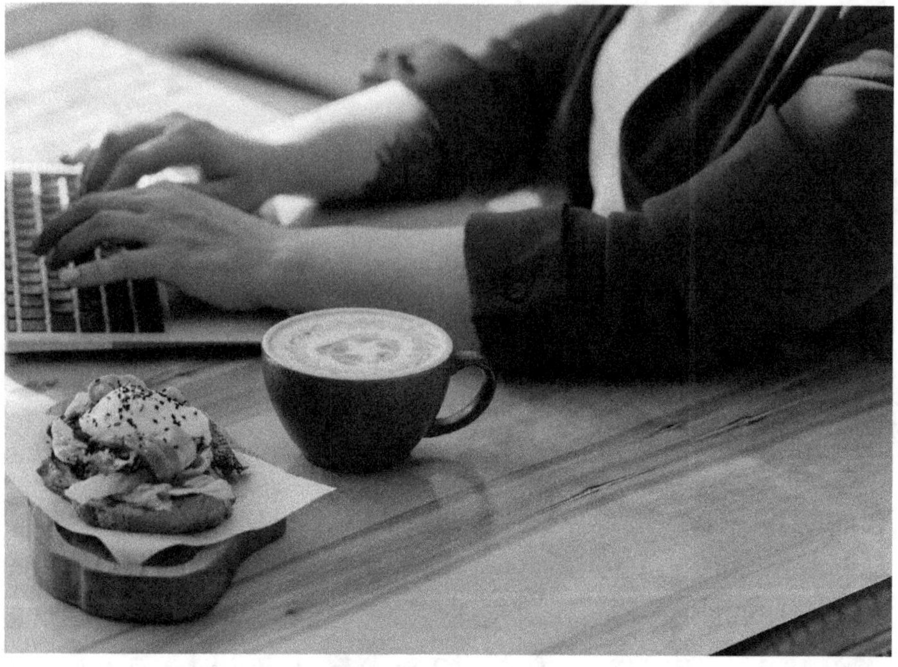

Sedentary lifestyle and poor nutrition contribute significantly to the increase in obesity. The opportunities for physical activity have been reduced by the introduction of technological instruments such as elevators, cars and remote controls. We spend more time on sedentary activities, such as using the computer, watching television and playing video games. In addition, the types of work have become more sedentary. Work in the office or at the desk has replaced manual work. Those who lead a sedentary lifestyle need fewer calories than more active people and therefore require a diet with a lower calorie intake. If the latter is not reduced, weight is gained.

Stereotypes society

It is a new society today, a 2.0 society, of self-care and self-diagnosis. A society in which stereotypes and prejudices are the masters, especially with regards to external beauty. Today, in fact, a body is defined as beautiful only when it is able to wear tight sizes and trendy clothes.

All this has consequences. To look beautiful, you need to be online and follow diets, most often found on websites or by famous people who promote their healthy diet. Strange diets, accompanied by supplements and pseudo-drugs that guarantee excellent results in a short time. Diets that through a few steps, can be found and available to everyone, without being calibrated on the person, without particular medical visits and without being prescribed by specialists in the sector.

Contentment and satisfaction for one's body have always been topics treated and considered almost an obsession. In the beginning, this was mainly visible in the female. Today, however, it seems that the male world has adopted these nuances, but in a different way. The lack of fulfillment for males focuses on a lack or lack of muscles or poorly defined physicality. In women it focuses on thinness or elimination of fat mass. In fact, for these and other reasons, eating disorders such as Bulimia, Anorexia, Vomiting and Binge Eating mainly affect the female population, even if there are significant exceptions.

Eating disorders are described as pathologies characterized by alterations in eating habits and by excessive concern about one's image, in particular weight and body shapes.

Social Reactions

Social reactions to obese people are often negative. The obese arouses anger. A social weight appears, surrounded by depressing prejudices like a greedy, lazy being, without self-control. Often people avoid sitting nearby on public transport. Comedians don't feel the need to hold back in their jokes. We imagine that in the near future the obese will be able to consider themselves subject to discrimination and believe they are stalking victims. And that the word fat will be considered politically incorrect.

Even in past, a limited number of obese did not represent a social problem, nor require health policy interventions. Indeed, people in the flesh enjoyed a particular social prestige and their body mass inspired confidence, as well as representing, in some eras, an ideal of beauty.

Since then, psychology has taken matters into its own hands. Together with the natural and anthropometric sciences, which give normality increasingly exact weights, shapes and volumes. And at the same time the language also creates neologisms to define in an ever more detailed way those intermediate states between fat and thin that previously had no name. Diminutive and augmentative, such as plump, rotund, fleshed, corpulent, plump, fat, which are in fact personal words, calibrating judgments.

These over sizes are the pariahs of the global village. First, I took my throat from the planetary junk food market, of which they are the insatiable financiers. And then stigmatized by a system that points to public condemnation as compulsive omnivores, unproductive parasites, unwilling subjects, time bombs for the health system, unsustainable overweight for welfare. How to say humiliated and obese. And also punished.

So much so that they earn on average eighteen percent less than normal weight. This is shown, figures in hand, by a recent Swedish research. However, obesity is not a disease that strikes at random regardless of eating habits and lifestyle.

Food Ignorance

In industrialized countries, nutrition consists of foods that contain many calories in a relatively small amount. Most of these foods contain a higher amount of refined carbohydrates and fats, and a lower amount of fiber.

Ready-made foods, such as high-calorie snacks available at vending machines and fast-food restaurants, contribute to the increase in obesity. High-calorie drinks, including sodas, juices, many coffee-based drinks and alcohol, also contribute significantly.

Larger portions served in restaurants and prepackaged food and drinks encourage you to consume too much food. In addition, the foods served in restaurants and packaged ones often have high-calorie preparations, therefore, it is possible that you consume a large amount of calories without realizing it.

Food hurts when we ingest too much and too often, and then because a large part of the food we ingest is bad, not genuine, adulterated, sophisticated. A person who consciously feeds on good food will not tend to obesity. By good food we mean moderate portions, homemade preparations starting from simple and poorly treated ingredients, eating at least once a day, at regular times sitting at a table and possibly in company.

Consuming good food is avoiding buying in the supermarket and offering children as calming packs of bottles of sweet and carbonated drinks, preserved and sugary fruit juices, elaborate packaged products such as chips, snacks and sweets.

Critical Consumption of Food

Across the western world, but not only, the growth in the percentage of obese people is increasingly dramatic. The consequence of their condition is to become seriously ill. If the main culprits of overweight have been identified for some time in Junk food and carbonated drinks, a serious information campaign to avert the danger has not yet been started.

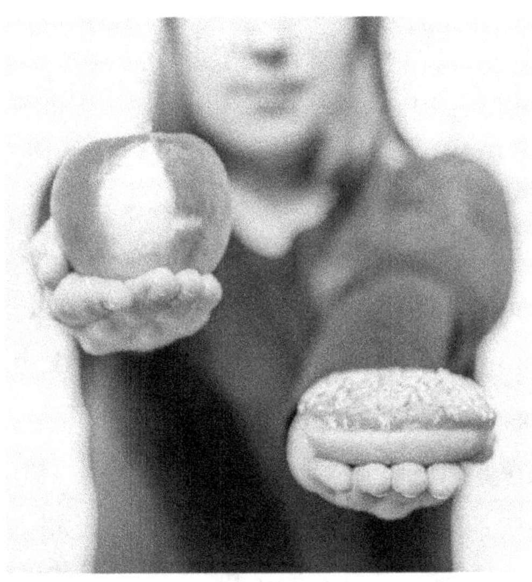

Many people still have not understood how genuine food choices can represent the only real protection against heart attacks, hypertension, stroke, diabetes and therefore be a guarantee of health and longevity. If the institutions provided information on the link between the so-called wellness diseases, hypertension, diabetes, cardiovascular problems and a diet rich in meat and dairy products, a gradual change in lifestyle and the burden of health costs would be induced. The public would shrink.

It would be appropriate to introduce the teaching of notions of nutrition and healthy and genuine gastronomy in the didactic programs. However, the resistance to such a radical change is still very strong, both from public opinion and from institutions, thanks to the very powerful industrial food lobbies,

The truth is that we are still tied to the myth of the flesh, to the idea that it is indispensable. Concepts and prejudices that are as entrenched as they are wrong. We eat meat thinking that it is the basis of nourishment. A steak provides protein and iron, but in equal if not less quantities than legumes. In addition it contains cholesterol and saturated fats, totally absent from the vegetable option.

Then, it is appropriate to reiterate that too often people forget that today we eat chickens built in the laboratory, modified in DNA. Their meats are 3 times fatter than those of old chickens and imbued with toxic substances deriving from antibiotics and hormones administered to chickens in large quantities and irresponsibly. Public canteens should provide for the introduction of an option as an alternative to dishes containing animal products or ingredients.

However, most doctors still claim the usefulness of feeding on meat. When they prescribe a diet they do not eliminate it but they prescribe lean meat, without sauces, without fats. While generally when eating meat, for the sake of the taste of the palate, we eat very seasoned meat, many sausages, chops. Nobody eats unseasoned chicken. Only those who are on a diet, in fact. But when it comes to eating meat, we are not talking about uncooked chicken, but more tasty and fatty meat. However, given the proven huge environmental impact of meat, the problem will have to be addressed. It is not possible to go ahead and take resources from the planet just to satisfy the palate.

Consequently, it is appropriate for the medical world, in a more scientific and objective way, to affirm that cereals, legumes, vegetables and fruit are able to provide the necessary for our organism a balanced nutritional intake.

Keep an eye on the food we eat, be careful, this seems to be the warning to follow. It is important to also keep in mind our environmental footprint, i.e. the production of greenhouse gases and the indiscriminate and increasingly unsustainable withdrawal of resources water, land, from the planet, by the meat industry. People need to be offered the diets they need to lead healthy lives, to fight obesity and being overweight, especially in countries that import most of their food. Excessive consumption of highly processed and high salt, sodium, sugars and trans fats imported foods is the main trigger of this situation. Estimates indicate that today 2.6 billion people are overweight and that the prevalence of obesity in the world population increased from 11.7 percent in 2012 to 13.2 percent in 2019.

If we don't take urgent action to stop the growth in obesity rates, we will soon have more obese people than undernourished in the world. There are several factors that favor this global obesity pandemic, and unhealthy diets are among the most significant.

First of all, there is the increased availability and ease of access to highly energetic foods rich in fats, sugars and salt, whose sales have been favored by intense advertising and marketing campaigns.

Fast-food and junk food are the best examples of this. This type of food is cheaper and easier to access than fresh food, especially for the poorest in urban areas. When resources for food start to run low, people choose cheaper foods, often high in calories but low in nutrients.

The Front of Food

Therefore on the food front there is a battle between itself and the world, between nature and culture. The struggle between control and impulsivity, between health and disease, is fought. On the food front, there are borders, limits and possibilities, between subjectivity and social relationship. In this context, many individual strategies compensating for our contradictions find space and many of the anxieties that are being generated are channeled.

The food front is also an extreme defense. In a world where you can no longer control anything, where you have lost all certainty and the possibility of self-determination, it is easy to fall into the trap of hyper-control. Through diet, it may happen that an attempt is made to restore a sort of existential balance that one feels he has lost.

Food restriction, brought to its extreme consequences, can lead to anorexia. Conversely, food overabundance, brought to its extreme consequences can lead to bulimia, obesity and binge-eating-disorder.

Critical food consumption is capable of regaining a balancing dimension, understood as a critical exercise on controlling the quality and quantity of food, which one feels to have lost.

The risk is that the battle to achieve proper nutrition produces an ever wider barrier between the self and the world. It is possible to restore a right relationship with food, in a world that produces overabundance but also food risk. The answer to this question needs a multidisciplinary perspective that sees the contribution of sociologists, psychologists, psychiatrists, anthropologists and experts in the field.

However, scientific research has taken many steps in recent years and models have been created to understand which pathways lead to disease and which factors increase the risk of getting sick.

2. EATING BEHAVIOR DISORDERS

Eating disorders are pathologies characterized by an alteration of eating habits and by an excessive concern for weight and body shapes.

They affect all people of all ages. They arise mainly during adolescence, especially female, with regard to certain pathologies such as anorexia and bulimia.

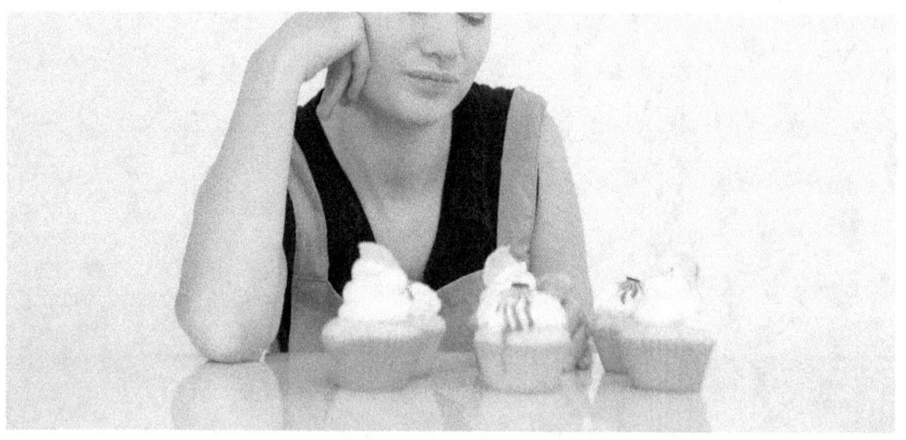

The typical behaviors of an eating disorder are revealed with the decrease in food intake, with fasting and bulimic crises. A significant amount of food is ingested in a short period of time, vomiting, the use of anorectic agents, laxatives are used and intense physical activity is used, in order to control weight.

Some people may resort to one or more of these behaviors, but this does not necessarily mean that they suffer from an eating disorder. There are in fact very specific diagnostic criteria that clarify what is to be understood as pathological.

Suffering from an eating disorder upsets a person's life and limits his or her relationship, work and social skills. For the person suffering from an eating disorder everything revolves around food and the fear of gaining weight. Things that once seemed trivial now become difficult and cause for anxiety.

Thoughts about food often haunt the person even when he is not at the table, for example at school or at work. Completing a task can become very difficult because in the head there seems to be room only for thoughts on what to eat, on the fear of gaining weight or having a bulimic crisis.

Only a small percentage of people suffering from an eating disorder ask for help. Sometimes people get complimented during their initial weight loss and this can reinforce the feeling of doing the right thing. On the other hand, when things start to worry, for the exaggerate weight loss or otherwise, it involves an important change in the person. This could start a panic crisis.

Generally, it is the family members who, first of all, alarmed by excessive weight loss, realize that something is wrong. Even for them, however, it is not easy to interfere, especially when the daughter or son does not yet have any awareness of the problem.

Not recognizing that you have a problem or using the symptoms of an eating disorder to try to solve your difficulties can have important consequences on requesting treatment.

An almost always present feature in those suffering from an eating disorder is the alteration of the body image which can become a real disorder. The perception that the person has of his own appearance or the way in which the idea of his body and forms was formed in his mind, seem to influence his life more than his real image.

Often the eating disorder is associated with other psychiatric diseases, in particular depression, but also anxiety disorders, alcohol or substance abuse, obsessive-compulsive disorder and personality disorders. Self-attacking behaviors may be present, such as self-injurious acts, such as scratching or cutting oneself up to obtain small injuries, burning parts of the body, and suicide attempts. This type of ailments occupy a very particular area in the field of psychiatry, since in addition to affecting the mind and therefore causing intense mental suffering, they also involve the body with sometimes very serious physical complications.

The main eating disorders are anorexia, bulimia, obesity and binge-eating-disorder, BED.

Anorexia

The term anorexia derives from the Greek "anorexia" and literally means lack of appetite. However, this is not an entirely appropriate definition, as the central node of anorexia is not the fact of not feeling hungry but a pathological desire to be thin.

Anorexia consists in the loss or reduction of appetite. The anorexic person despite being slim and having a weight lower than the values considered normal continues not to accept his body always seeing himself as fat.

Poor nutrition or even the resulting fasting can cause serious damage to the endocrine system leading to the absence of menstruation in women with serious consequences for fertility or increasing the risk of heart disease and osteoporosis. It mainly affects the female sex in the adolescent bracket.

For those who drop below 40 kg, they risk death from heart complications. Obviously, anorexia should not be seen only as an aesthetic dislike but must be considered an internal malaise. People suffering from anorexia nervosa are therefore underweight due to a strong decrease in food intake.

Those suffering from Anorexia often do not realize their thinness, rather they are terrified of the idea of gaining weight and becoming fat. They try to have a very strict discipline on the control of food and one's weight. People with Anorexia also give excessive weight and body shapes to assess themselves, as if their self-esteem depended on being thin and being able to control their diet.

Another feature of Anorexia in women is amenorrhea, that is, the lack of the menstrual cycle for at least three consecutive months due to weight loss and food restriction. Even when the person regains weight in some cases it takes some time before the menstrual cycle returns to being regular.

Often the disease can begin gradually and sneakily. For example, a girl can start eating a little less for different reasons.

She may lose a few extra pounds, for general digestive problems, physical ailments or surgery. It is common for the onset of the disorder to be preceded by stressful events or by important changes in life or residence, breakdown of a romantic relationship or school difficulties.

There are two different forms of anorexia, one defined as "restrictive" in which weight loss and control are due to fasting, food restriction and sometimes excessive physical activity.

Other defined compensation behaviors are characterized by the presence of bulimic crisis, together with fasting, and have the purpose of decreasing body weight. Self-induced vomiting can come through the use of improper use of diuretics or laxatives.

These two forms also differ from a psychological point of view. The restrictive form is often characterized by rigidity, obstinacy, perfectionism and obsessive-compulsive spectrum disorders and has a more favorable prognosis. The bulimic-purgative form is often accompanied by intense psychic discomfort, depression and impulsive behavior.

Bulimia

Bulimia, literally "ox hunger", is characterized by the presence of bulimic or binge crises, followed by compensatory behaviors aimed at hindering weight gain.

To reach a diagnosis of Bulimia Nervosa all the following diagnostic criteria, DSM 5 Diagnostic and Statistical Manual of Mental Disorders, must be present.

You eat more food in a certain period of time than most people would eat at the same time. You have the feeling that you are unable to stop eating or to control what and how much you are eating, followed by binge eating compensatory behaviors. Recurrent and inappropriate compensatory behaviors are used to prevent weight gain, such as self-induced vomiting, abuse of laxatives, diuretics or other drugs, fasting or excessive physical activity. Self-esteem levels are unduly influenced by the shape and weight of the body.

Bulimia Nervosa

Some people think they are bulimic because they think they overeat. In reality, the bulimic crisis, whose fundamental characteristic is Bulimia Nervosa, has very specific criteria. Thinking of exaggerating with a few more slices of dessert or ice cream certainly does not represent a real bulimic crisis.

A binge falls within the diagnostic criteria for Bulimia, when the person eats an objectively abundant amount of food in a given period of time, 1-2 hours, having the feeling of losing control and not being able to stop.

Usually the binges are made with foods considered prohibited such as sweets, carbohydrates and fats, foods that outside of binges, people with Bulimia try to eliminate from their diet. Bulimic crises must occur at least twice a week.

There are two subtypes of bulimia, the purgative and the non-purgative one. The purgative form is characterized by the presence of elimination conduits such as self-induced vomiting, by the improper use of diuretics, laxatives or enemas. Vomiting can be induced through mechanical stimulation of the throat or through the ingestion of fluids or compression of the stomach.

In the non-purgative form, the compensation methods are fasting or excessive exercise, but vomiting or other forms of purgative compensation are not regularly present. All compensatory behaviors, in any form, interfere and significantly condition the lives of people suffering from this disorder.

People with Bulimia Nervosa usually have a normal weight, although in some cases they may be overweight. A very important factor in the onset of Bulimia Nervosa is diet.

Often those who suffer from Bulimia outside of binges try to follow a very restricted diet, starting an alternating cycle of diet and bulimic crisis that consolidates and maintains the disorder itself. In some cases, bulimic crises, a low-calorie diet, follow a set of unpleasant sensations and emotions such as loneliness, boredom, anger. These are all tensions that the person manages with difficulty.

Psychological Characteristics

Often the onset of Bulimia occurs following a low-calorie diet or following a stressful event or a real emotional trauma. If at first the bulimic crisis can be occasional or occasional over time it becomes a compulsion that is difficult to escape.

In Bulimia Nervosa, attention and dissatisfaction with one's body and physical aspect can assume absolute importance. Self-esteem is strongly linked to the body and any physical modification can be experienced as a frustration and as a loss of control over one's body.

The emotional consequences of a binge can be different. In some cases, people report experiencing temporary relief and a sense of pleasure. As in most of the eating disorders in which bulimic crises are found, usually these erroneously positive effects are soon replaced by a deep anguish for the possibility of gaining weight and because you have not managed to control yourself. Compensation methods, especially vomiting, can give the temporary sensation of alleviating anxiety but afterwards a sense of emptiness may appear which in turn can trigger a new binge.

An almost always present feeling is that of shame and guilt. And this is why the disease is often hidden from family and friends for as long as possible and in many cases the request for help is made after a long time after the trouble has started.

Bulimia Nervosa not only changes eating habits, but also other important areas of the person's life. It can happen to give up the social situations that involve being at the table with others, or to become anxious and irritable and make relationships with others very difficult and tense.

Bulimia Nervosa is often associated with other mental disorders such as depression, such as substance abuse, anxiety disorders, social phobia, obsessive compulsive disorder, panic disorder and personality disorders. It is not uncommon for self-aggressive behavior such as suicide attempts or self-harming acts to occur.

Psychologically affected people with bulimia nervosa exhibit certain characteristics such as perfectionism. Often it is expressed in the imposition of very high levels of expectation both in daily life and in the objectives related to nutrition. Anything that deviates from absolute success is considered a failure and can weaken a very low and vulnerable self-esteem in most of the times.

The "all or nothing" thought is expressed with the tendency to see things in black or white, to divide them into good or bad. The food will then be good or dangerous, a day will be either totally positive or catastrophic. The bulimic crisis is often triggered by all or nothing thinking. The person, convinced that he has now transgressed the iron diet, after eating even small quantities of food, guided by thought, so much so that they have ruined everything, continues in the binge.

Low self-esteem aggravates this aspect of personality. Losing control over the diet in a binge can result in depression, disappointment and anguish. The fact of not being able to maintain a strict diet and indeed having distorted it from bulimic crises makes bulimic patients feel unworthy, guilty and worthless.

In some cases, in Bulimia Nervosa there may be considerable difficulty in controlling and managing impulses. Often they can manifest themselves with behaviors such as making small cuts or burns on the skin, adopting promiscuous sexual behavior, using alcohol or drugs, putting themselves in dangerous situations.

Medical Complications

The physical complications of Bulimia Nervosa are related to compensatory behaviors. Vomiting and improper use of laxatives and diuretics can cause various physical complications. Frequent vomiting can have serious consequences. It can cause an electrolyte imbalance, i.e. a modification of body fluids and electrolytes, such as sodium and potassium.

The most serious complication is hypokalaemia, a reduction in the level of potassium. It can cause hypochloremia and changes in heart rhythm, up to cardiac arrest. The most frequent symptoms of an electrolyte imbalance are dizziness, thirst, water retention, fatigue and apathy. These changes are reversible and disappear when the person stops vomiting. Loss of gastric juice through vomiting can lead to metabolic alkalosis and metabolic acidosis. Vomiting in the long run irreversibly erodes the tooth enamel, especially the inside of the front teeth. In some people who induce vomiting there is an enlargement of the salivary glands. It may happen that the swelling of the glands causes an enlargement of the face, which may suggest that the body has also enlarged, increasing the concern for the weight and body shape.

Reflux esophagitis is a medical condition characterized by the presence of lesions of the esophageal mucosa secondary to retrograde reflux of gastric contents. In people who use their fingers to induce vomiting, small wounds may be present above the knuckles of the hand, initially they are abrasions and then become scars. The mechanical stimulation of vomiting can cause superficial wounds in the back of the throat that can lead to infections. Sore throats and hoarseness are frequent. Vomiting can rarely cause lacerations or bleeding to the esophagus. However, if a certain amount of fresh blood appears in the vomit, a medical examination should be immediately requested to exclude a laceration in the stomach.

Obesity

Obesity is a chronic disease caused by an excess of fat mass distributed differently in the various body areas. To talk about obesity, excess weight must exceed 20% of the ideal weight for height. The simplest and most used parameter to define the degree of obesity is the Body Mass Index and height.

Obesity is not defined univocally. The common orientation is that above a certain body weight it should be considered a chronic pathology like diabetes or high blood pressure. Obese subjects appear to have a reduced life expectancy and a quality of the same compromised.

The adolescent period constitutes a delicate moment for the obese subject. About 75% of cases are a condition that begins before six years of age. However the symptoms occur at any age.

Overweight is perceived as a lack of will, gluttony, little regard for one's health and aesthetics. They use the consumer-food item as an illusory promise to replace the vacuum, but without obtaining anything, just satisfaction. The obese subject accumulates within himself an unlimited amount of food until he feels suffocated.

The body is a prison, it is not felt as one's own, and this armor serves as a shield, as a paradoxical defense against the demands of the other. There is an attempt to anesthetize emotions through an apparent physical enjoyment.

In filling up with everything, one does not experience the emptiness which is what produces thought, desire, and creative acts. The fullness tries to fill the anguish of the void, but it leads to the anguish of a fullness that suffocates and cancels the subject.

Advices for those who suffer from Obesity

Obesity does not pose a direct threat to the life of the individual, except in cases where there is an excess of weight greater than 60%. Certainly, however, it is still compromising the quality of life of the subjects affected. Indirectly it can cause death, since it involves a whole series of serious medical complications.

The currently applicable therapeutic measures must elicit active patient participation in order to be truly effective. Obviously, this participation must be motivated by the recognition of a dissatisfaction linked to the malaise experienced before and after binge eating. It could be boredom, loneliness, the depressive void, which often follows the act of eating, and aesthetic concerns.

This awareness often occurs in adolescence, when the motivation for change is so high that it leads to a greater probability of success. This change does not take place by resorting to a DIY restrictive diet. It is widely recognized that the restriction is a cause of loss of control and therefore of binge eating. This entails a vicious circle of failures that feed low self-esteem, shame, depression, inability to control oneself.

It is necessary to contact a specialist, or better yet a specialized center in which a program that goes beyond the diet is implemented. It is important to look at the person with their experiences, their beliefs, and possibly act on a psychological, educational and behavioral level.

Psychotherapy and Obesity

A serious treatment of obesity should be based both on an assessment of eating behavior and on a cognitive-behavioral program.

Long-term success will be more likely if weight loss will result from a change in lifestyle and dysfunctional behaviors that determine the establishment and maintenance of obesity.

The weight loss diet alone is more likely to recur, with the regaining of the lost pounds, 90-95% of cases. Instead, the goal must be to achieve and maintain a modest but manageable weight loss to improve health conditions.

For this reason, the treatment should also include an educational program aimed at changing eating behavior, promoting motor activity and changing body weight.

The patient should be actively involved in all phases of therapy, informed, educated, supported as in a rehabilitation process. The drastic diet inevitably leads to loss of control with a consequent unscheduled or controlled calorie intake.

Instead, the goal is precisely the acquisition of the ability to control itself, which is achieved by replacing the rigid control with a schedule that also provides for the previously programmed transgression. By managing the diet you are able to experience the pleasantness of control.

Feeling the pleasure of being able to control yourself allows you to get out of failures and guilt. It is a long, difficult path, but possible through the management of a program entrusted to multiple operators who take care of the person as a whole.

Pharmacological therapy and Obesity

To complete the discussion, it seems appropriate to specify that obesity therapy often involves the administration of drugs. Clearly we are talking about particularly serious cases, above all of a mere support to the therapeutic measures exposed so far, which represent the cornerstone of the cure. The drugs used belong to three classes, of the thyroid hormones, diuretics, psychotropics and anorexants. Obviously the use of do-it-yourself is strongly discouraged. The drugs must be administered only under strict medical supervision, also because their uncontrolled intake can lead to very serious damage.

3. BINGE EATING DISORDER

The Binge Eating Disorder, BED, is a disorder characterized by the presence of bulimic crises in the absence of inappropriate compensation behaviors for weight control.

People with Binge Eating Disorder are rarely recognized. They are mistakenly confused with other overweight or obese people, or worse with bulimic ones.

Even those who suffer from uncontrolled eating disorder experience a sense of shame and dissatisfaction with their body, even if an ideal of extreme thinness is not necessarily pursued. They feel a deep sense of discomfort in losing control with food, but unlike obese subjects, they give excessive weight or body figure to assess themselves.

What is the Binge Eating Disorder?

The Binge Eating Disorder, BED is the eating disorder characterized by recurrent episodes of binge eating always accompanied by a feeling of loss of weight control.

Compared to other patients with eating disorders, subjects with uncontrolled feeding disorder have on average a greater weight, a greater frequency of overweight or obesity. Often people with Binge Eating Disorder visit the centers for the treatment of obesity, but compared to patients with obesity they report a greater presence of psychiatric symptoms, in particular depression, anxiety and personality disorders.

Those who suffer from Binge Eating Disorder experienced a sense of shame and dissatisfaction with their body, even if an ideal of extreme thinness is not necessarily pursued. They feel a deep sense of discomfort in losing control with food, but they do not always give excessive weight or body figure to assess themselves. Like people with obesity, people with BED can be discriminated against by others because of their physical condition.

Those with this eating disorder feel dissatisfied, lacking self-esteem, disgusted with themselves and depressed. In certain very serious cases, the pathology of uncontrolled feeding disorder degenerates into cases of self-harm and instinct to suicide.

Debut of the Binge Eating Disorder

Binge Eating Disorder is a disorder that shares some psychopathological aspects with other eating disorders and is almost always associated with obesity. The study of the subject's personality with BED appears useful to etiology science, the sector that deals with researching the causes of the phenomena. In recent decades, numerous researches have stimulated many questions for which further studies are required to provide the appropriate answers. Generally speaking, these are studies on why certain events or processes occur and on the reasons behind certain events.

Binge Eating Disorder typically begins in adolescence or early adulthood, but can also begin in late adulthood. It can appear at any age, affects both genders, with a greater prevalence in male persons. Those affected by it come to the attention of the clinician usually later than individuals with nervous bulimia. Often it is not associated with an emotional discomfort and a diet is usually required as a first intervention, after the numerous and often unsuccessful DIY diets.

In patients with Binge Eating Disorders often, incongruous diets or their failure represent the event that triggers a binge. In this case, however, it is the negative emotions related to the deprivation of the pleasure of food or to the finding of the difficulty in losing weight to induce to exceed in nutrition. Intolerance to negative emotions is definitely an important psychopathological construct for this disorder.

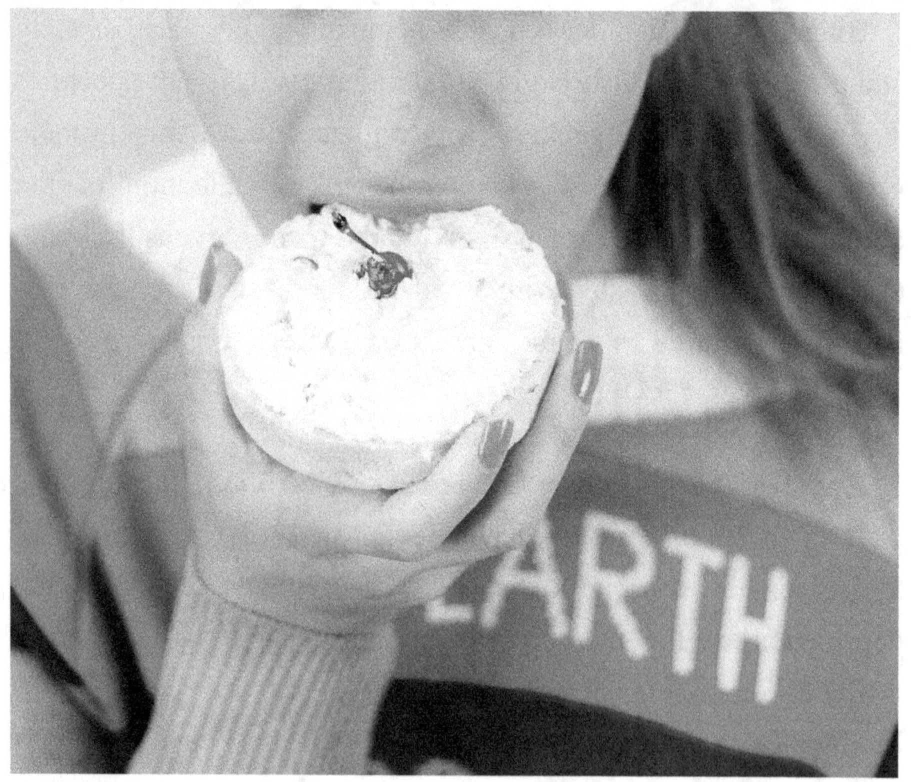

It appears to be recurrent in families, which may reflect genetic influences. There are several studies on risk factors and binge triggers, but none offer completely comprehensive answers. It should be underlined, however, the fact that in addition to genetic factors, neuroendocrine and social factors also appear to be involved. The difficult experiences of childhood life, the presence of depressive disorders in the parents, the tendency to obesity and the repeated exposure to negative comments regarding the form, weight and mode of feeding would seem to play a central role for a reliable diagnosis.

The disorder by BEG occurs in normal weight, overweight and obese individuals. In binge eating, binges are not followed by elimination or compensation practices such as vomiting or purges. Those who have been suffering from it for a long time or in a serious way are unavoidable to experience overweight or obesity. Beyond the psychic discomfort that the person suffering from BED is experiencing, the obesity or overweight condition he may experience will also lead to cardiological, respiratory disorders, typical of obesity.

Developing phases of the Binge Eating Disorder

Individuals with Binge Eating Disorder feed differently than obese or bulimic patients. It is the attitude towards food that is different in these patients. For them, food is an uncomfortable ally, capable of consoling in the saddest moments and gratifying in those of joy, which at the same time leaves behind the guilt of the binge and an unpleasant residue of unnecessary pounds.

A peculiar characteristic of the subject affected is represented by the behavior after the binge. It does not take an active attitude, aimed at restoring the antecedent state, but the passivity, discouragement and sense of inevitability of one's destiny prevails. There is almost never an attempt to remedy the incident that goes beyond good intentions, destined to be regularly disregarded. This attitude is closer to the attitude of a depressed patient than one suffering from eating disorders.

It often emerges that people with uncontrolled eating disorder experience greater levels of anxiety and depression, as well as greater dissatisfaction with their bodies. However, sometimes Binge Eating Disorder patients report binge eating even after positive emotions. The inability to manage emotions leads to excess in uncontrolled nutrition. Binge eating thus becomes the final common response to different emotions, to more disparate moments and events, capable of soothing any discomfort.

An episode of binge eating is defined as eating significantly more food over a certain period of time than most individuals would eat at the same time and in similar circumstances. An episode of excessive consumption of food must be accompanied by the feeling of losing control to be considered a binge episode. These binge episodes are normally characterized by marked discomfort.

Diagnostic criteria of the BED

Those affected by BED implement a series of behaviors that act as clear alarm bells. People suffering from this eating disorder tend to binge or ingest a significant amount of food very quickly. Many patients eat large quantities of food even if they do not feel absolutely hungry and, often and willingly, eat meals alone for the shame of showing up in public.

An episode of uncontrolled feeding is characterized by the presence of two factors:

☐ Eat, in a defined period of time, for example two hours, a quantity of food that is decidedly greater than what most people would eat in the same period of time and in the same circumstances;

☐ Feel a feeling that you can't stop eating and can't control what and how much you eat.

Uncontrolled Feeding Episodes

The most frequent symptoms to be able to establish that it is a diagnosis of a disorder are due to the fact of eating large quantities of food much faster than normal to feel unpleasantly full. Eating alone because of the embarrassment of how much you are eating and feeling disgusted with yourself, depressed and guilty about yourself.

Uncontrolled nutrition is not associated with the systematic use of inappropriate compensatory behaviors, such as the use of laxatives, self-induced vomiting, fasting or physical hyperactivity. A key feature is the loss of control during the episode which however varies between people. Some warn themselves long before they start eating, for others there is a gradual evolution and for still others it comes only after they realize they have eaten too much.

There is a close relationship between BED and obesity. In fact, most people with this disorder are obese or overweight. This does not mean, however, that all obese people are affected by Binge Eating Disorder.

Psychological Characteristics

Compared to other patients with eating disorders, people suffering from BED appear to be less symptomatic. Although, compared with other obese patients who do not have an eating disorder, BEDs report greater psychiatric symptoms, in particular depression, anxiety and personality disorders.

They feel a deep sense of discomfort in losing control over food, but they do not always place excessive importance on weight or body figure to evaluate themselves. Often, people with this disorder are teased and discriminated against by others. It is generally thought that their overweight or obesity is due to excessive gluttony and lack of control.

People suffering from BED are aware that their weight is not only a matter of will, but there are important genetic implications. On the other hand, their almost always irregular diet leads them to feel guilty of their own weight and to live with a deep sense of shame. The more frequent bulimic seizures are, the more people with BED may feel depressed and exhibit other psychiatric symptoms. It therefore seems that the weight, the bulimic crises and the mood tone interact with each other, promoting dysfunctional maintenance of the disorder itself.

BED and the Psychobiological Model of Personality

In order to understand the Binge Eating Disorder well, it is interesting to refer to the psychobiological model of the personality. It could prove to be an additional key to understanding the disorder itself and could help explain such a peculiar disorder.

According to this approach there are temperamental and character dimensions, which could constitute a specific personality model of the BED.

In particular, a high activity of Novelty Seeking NS, exploratory factor of the sphere of impulsiveness and aggression, rewards a rapid loss of anger and avoiding the consequent frustration, in avoiding the damage, would correspond to an anxious-depressive spectrum.

On the contrary, a low activity of Self Directness, SD, corresponds to an indicator of fragility, a difficulty in containing a temperament characterized by impulsiveness and a predisposition to develop a personality disorder.

Impulsiveness and compulsiveness, the pillars of the personality of these patients, are the basis of various dysfunctional behaviors. Such features are present, for example, in the diagnosis of borderline and antisocial personality disorder, attention deficit or hyperactivity disorder, impulse control disorders.

From a clinical point of view, the low activity of Self Directness could prove very useful for drawing up a psychotherapeutic project for its treatment.

Characteristics of the BED

The disease is characterized by an alteration of eating habits and by an excessive concern for weight and body shapes. The medical complications observed in patients with BED are generally related to the presence of obesity, such as cardiovascular, metabolic problems, such as diabetes and dyslipidema, osteo-articular, gastric-intestinal, respiratory, and difficulty healing from wounds.

The evolution of the BED is little known because of its too recent definition and characterization. Some researchers say that the cure rates are similar to those of Bulimia Nervosa that is about 57%, even if these data need further investigation.

An almost always present feature in those suffering from an eating disorder is the alteration of the body image which can become a real disorder. The perception that the person has of his appearance seems to influence his life more than his real image. The body becomes the theater of a profound suffering experienced by the subject. It is the body that must communicate. The image that refers to the mirror is in their eyes that of a person with too wide hips, with too large thighs and with too large a belly. The evaluation of oneself, in subjects suffering from other eating disorders, depends excessively by the weight and shape of your body. The body becomes the bearer of traumatic, difficult and unbearable experiences.

The Role of Impulsiveness

Binge eating occurs, on average, at least once a week and patients experience difficulties in various areas of their lives. First of all, they feel a sort of social unease, extended to most interpersonal relationships. They perceive a distortion in the vision of their body which feeds a sense of insecurity and inadequacy. They register a certain pressure and stress due to the large amount of time spent on a diet and in some cases, they resort to alcohol or drug abuse. They have difficulty managing moods or expressing their emotions, including anger. Their sense of helplessness is linked to the inability to control their eating behavior and the consequent weight gain.

Compared to other patients with eating disorders, subjects suffering from BED have an average weight, a greater frequency of overweight or obesity.

However, compared to patients with obesity, they report a greater presence of psychiatric symptoms, in particular depression, anxiety and personality disorders. Like people with obesity, people with BEG can be discriminated against by others because of their physical condition.

They feel a deep sense of discomfort in losing control with food, but unlike people with bulimia nervosa, they do not always give excessive weight or body figure to assess themselves.

50% of patients with BEG suffer from major depression, panic disorder and some personality disorders. In fact, the binge eating symptom would compensate for a pervasive sensation of persistent discomfort present at the time of the crisis. A high overweight can contribute to the maintenance and accentuation of the compulsive symptom. It gives back to those who suffer from it a sense of failure, guilt and shame that supports uncontrolled food behavior. During the binge episodes the subject is unaware of what he is doing, so there is a loss of control. Afterwards, they are prey to feelings of disgust.

Personality characteristics of the patients are considered as individual vulnerability factors. They allow those who are carriers of it to be more exposed than others to develop this disorder. The consideration of pathological personality traits in BEDs highlights the problem of co-morbidity, or the association of two or more disorders in the same subject. These are the so-called complex cases of particular importance for both research and clinical practice.

At the clinical level, people who are often impulsive and emotionally unrestrained are observed. Eating disorder is an impulsive-compulsive attempt to regulate feelings perceived as intolerable. In particular, some patients report feelings of despair, an inability to tolerate stress and spasmodic research for an immediate feeling of gratification. The uncontrolled intake of food and its elimination thus constitutes and reinforces itself as a failed self-care.

Considering that this disorder has been recognized only recently, the literature on this topic is not very well known. However, some studies concerning personality have focused on the dimension of impulsivity - compulsiveness.

As can be observed in the disorders that are part of the obsessive-compulsive continuum, in the same way in BED, in order to avoid the emotion of anxiety, an impulse is implemented that can guarantee a fallacious feeling of well-being.

Being able to give in to the impulse, in fact, generates a kind of subjective pleasure even if its consequences can be extremely tearing. The person, therefore, perceives that he cannot resist the urge to eat. Before committing the act, the subject feels an increased sense of tension. Only while he commits the act and then eats, does he experience pleasure and gratification.

However, this mechanism triggers a vicious circle whereby, at a later time, negative experiences come to light that arise mostly in the form of senses of guilt and shame.

BED and Impulsivity

In any case, in general, eating disorders and impulsivity would seem to share the same biological basis. Just as eating disorders could be interpreted in a continuum of serotonergic dysfunction.

Serotonin is an amino acid, naturally produced by specialized cells of the intestine and is known as 5-HT. The effect of 5-HT depends on signaling to target cells on brain tissues. It conditions the mood and promotes feelings of well-being. It also impairs appetite, sleep cycles and pain perception.

In impulsive subjects it has been shown that there is an alteration of the metabolism of serotonin and a reduction in the activity of this neurotransmitter. Interestingly, high levels of 5HT would induce anorexic behavior and obsessive-compulsive behavior. While, low levels of 5HT would produce impulsive behaviors, with loss of control over eating behavior. Consequence that subjects affected by BED would lead to bulimic behavior.

According to the cognitive approach, the patient would be subject to repeated extremes in the judgment of himself and the environment. All black or all white, there is no middle ground. The lack of sufficient self-awareness facilitates the onset and maintenance of extreme behaviors. This produces the alternation of restrictions and binges, such as to re-propose to the individual their inability to lead a balanced existence. The result could be dangerous, since the sense of failure is strengthened even in the face of a small food relapse. In this way, the onset of guilt, the insinuation and the subsequent perpetuation of depressive symptoms is favored.

In particular, impulsivity plays an important role especially in maintaining dysfunctional behavior. Faced with a potential threat, the individual with a strong trait of impulsiveness does not seem to have the cognitive resources necessary to adequately assess the event and identify the most appropriate response. On the contrary, there is a high probability that aggressive behavior will take place to protect or avoid pain. It is a matter of implementing a sudden response in reaction to a stimulus coming from the external environment through a behavioral scramble. The subject uses food behavior as a protection strategy. The method used not only in BED but also in other eating disorders seems to be linked by a single common thread. Illusively, one tries to control and manage one's emotional experience in an attempt that seems to want to reactivate the body with food. In addition to the concomitant presence of addiction to alcohol and drugs, in some subjects with BED there are other behaviors related to impulsiveness such as sexual promiscuity, kleptomania, self-injurious behavior or suicide attempts.

In light of the foregoing, it is pointed out that some features and modalities could compromise the already difficult treatment of these patients. In particular, perfectionism and impulsiveness can affect the treatment of these ailments by hindering the therapeutic alliance.

Acceptance of One's Emotions

Dysfunctional emotional management is one of the main characteristics of eating disorders. The study of the emotional state of patients is a branch that needs to be deepened in order to deal with those who are affected by Binge Eating Disorder with the right competence.

From our analysis it is clear that, in order to effectively deal with the problem of the Binge Eating Disorder, it is necessary to intervene with a psychological path. This path must be aimed at increasing the ability to regulate the emotions of the subjects, starting primarily from the work on accepting their negative emotions.

If the individual denies the possibility of experiencing certain types of emotions, the fact of increasing the emotional awareness in themselves is absolutely insufficient for the solution of their problems. As long as they do not legitimize themselves in their feelings, in fact, their emotional recognition will be worth nothing.

Acceptance of emotions is the fundamental element in order to be able to activate functional regulation strategies, which are not based on compromise but, rather, on addressing and regulating the emotion in place managing the situation that generated it.

In this regard, it may be useful to propose, in a psychological intervention aimed at managing the Binge Eating Disorder that allows you to reach a greater awareness of the emotions you feel, through an attitude of listening to yourself. Accepting emotions through a non-judgmental attitude allows you to accept the experience as it is and evaluate it without stereotyped labels or commonplaces.

Through the possibility of learning to recognize one's own bodily signals, the ability to accept one's emotions is developed without judging them at any cost. This attitude would avoid having to resort to defensive escapes and self-injurious behavior. In this way, we move from an automatic reactivity to the implementation of a response that is more suited to the needs of subjects who show a dysfunctional relationship with food.

Anger and Negative Emotions

Another interesting aspect would be to investigate which emotions are more difficult to accept by subjects who exhibit Binge Eating Disorder behaviors. One of the emotions to highlight is definitely anger. The greatest difficulty in relating is anger, which characterizes subjects with a dysfunctional relationship with food. Anger is experienced as a negative emotion.

Anger is experienced as wrong and not socially acceptable. It cannot have a positive meaning. However, the difference between experiencing anger and engaging in angry behavior is not considered. In this way, one cannot perceive the evolutionary meaning of anger or even experience the specific emotion of anger. It is possible that this particular difficulty in relating to anger is due to external judgment, towards those who are experiencing this relational situation; experiencing anger would, in fact, more easily lead to behaviors that can be misjudged by others.

Being badly judged for an abnormal behavior means having to question one's amiability and validity as individuals. With a view to a future development of a research study, it would be interesting to evaluate the modification of the ability to regulate the emotions of the subjects affected by Binge Eating Disorder following a mainly psychological path. Everything must be based on the enhancement of emotional regulation skills to allow subjects to accept their emotions, whatever they are.

4. PREVENTION AND CAUSE OF THE BINGE EATING DISORDER

Prevention

Prevention includes all those health and non-health interventions that seek to reduce the onset, chronicity and negative consequences of those affected by Binge Eating Disorder.

Prevention interventions are usually divided according to the moment in which they act. Before the onset of the disease and at the first signs of symptoms. It allows an early identification of the subjects concerned, and this one is the most opportune moment to reduce or eliminate the risk factors.

When the disorder is full-blown, the prevention coincides with the treatment of the disorder itself, to prevent patients' possible physical and mental complications.

Primary Prevention

Many scholars have wondered if preventing eating disorders is possible. There are many questions about the possibility of prevention and the answers are not univocal. Numerous studies in the field of eating disorders and their possible causes have led to understanding that there is no single cause for these disorders. Many factors combine to predispose, precipitate and then perpetuate the disorder. These factors are of various types, genetic factors, socio-cultural factors, psychological factors, biological factors.

By definition, primary prevention is possible only when the etiological factors are known and modifiable. If it is possible to intervene on socio-cultural pressures, it is not possible to intervene on genetic factors. It is very important to understand whether primary prevention interventions reduce the incidence of eating disorders. Explaining to someone or a group of people what eating disorders are is even counterproductive and harmful.

Mechanisms of imitation and identification can trigger, as often these serious diseases are idealized. The same automatism is triggered by the testimony of people who have suffered from these problems. For this reason, it is good to be wary of preventive programs based only on information regarding these ailments.

On the contrary, many studies have instead found that interventions that stimulate discussion and the development of a greater critical sense towards the messages of the mass media can be useful. This type of intervention should not deal exclusively with eating disorders, but range more widely on the different problems of one's own experience, the relationships one has with one's body and interpersonal problems.

Other forms of potentially useful intervention could be interventions aimed at people at high risk, or interventions that aim to enhance protective factors, improve self-esteem, problem solving and communication skills.

It is therefore essential to evaluate the effectiveness of the preventive programs before implementing them. In times of rationalization of resources, it is important to invest in interventions of sure efficacy and without potential risks.

Secondary Prevention

Then there is another type of prevention, called secondary, which intervenes on cases as soon as possible with respect to the onset of the disorder. It has been ascertained, at a clinical level, that a treatment undertaken in the early stages of the disease is more effective. However, in the early stages of the disease, the person with an eating disorder does not always understand and admit that he needs help. Also at this level it is therefore important to raise awareness of the environment, starting from the same people interested in the family. The right prevention requires the ability to recognize eating disorders to facilitate the request for help in specialist centers, in general practitioners and specialists for these pathologies.

Food as a Relief from Negative Emotions

Compulsive nutrition is characterized by ingesting large quantities of pleasant foods, in order to alleviate a negative emotional state. This element can also be found, for example, in the symptoms of obsessive-compulsive disorder, from the decrease in the reward from anxiety and stress.

The diminished reward feature is characterized by the loss of motivation for ordinary rewards. The negative feeling derives from the involvement of the stress-related brain systems that are involved in this mechanism, causing irritability and anxiety.

Therefore, when a behavior becomes compulsive, a shift in the factors that motivated it is assumed. Initially the behavior is positively reinforced, later the compulsion could arise from the negative reinforcement mechanisms. Experiences of anxiety and irritability when the reward, that is, the food sought is not available, condition eating disorders that lead to compulsive eating behavior.

As regards nutrition, abstinence from certain foods is configured with a diet. It implies a reduction in the calories ingested, going from highly prohibited foods to an increase in healthier and less palatable foods. Numerous studies have in fact highlighted how the majority of obese subjects, at the beginning of the diet, experience intense sensations of irritability and anxiety. The transition from a food balance rich in calories to a less caloric one leads to a worsening of mood and depressive symptoms. Diet as a stress management strategy highlights that attempting emotional self-healing through comfort food is counterproductive.

The self-induced diet worsens a negative emotional state. Having access to palatable foods after a period of deprivation leads to excessive consumption. This alleviates the discomfort caused by depression and anxiety, but can lead to compulsive nutrition, instead of getting relief from anxiety or stress.

Negative Consequences of Compulsive Nutrition

The last element of compulsive nutrition seems to be the loss of control, due to a deficit in the mechanisms responsible for suppressing inappropriate actions. These deficits likely confer vulnerability to addictive behavior. Stakeholders are encouraged to delay dysfunctional behavior rather than end it.

This lack of inhibitory food control often persists despite the physical, psychological and social complications that lead to uncontrolled nutrition. These subjects often suffer from negative emotions following binges, due to experiences of shame, denial and guilt.

When these negative emotional and physical consequences outweigh the desirable effects of a pleasant food, people often attempt to start a diet, although they often fall back into improper and unhealthy eating habits.

Self-referential Company

It is a new society today, a 2.0 society, of self-care and self-diagnosis. A society in which stereotypes and prejudices are the masters, especially as to regards external beauty. Today, in fact, a body is defined as beautiful only when it is able to wear tight sizes and trendy clothes.

All this has consequences, to look beautiful, you have to be online and follow diets, most often found on websites or by famous people who promote their healthy diet.

Strange diets, accompanied by supplements and pseudo-drugs that guarantee excellent results in a short time. Diets that come from all over the world and that, through a few steps, can be found and available to everyone. The prescription of specialists who calibrate the diet on the person after an accurate medical examination is avoided.

Contentment and satisfaction for one's body have always been topics treated and considered as an obsession. In the beginning, this was mainly visible in the female sex, but today it seems that the male world has adopted this attitude too, but in a different way. The lack of fulfillment for males focuses on a lack or lack of muscles or poorly defined physicality. In women it focuses on thinness or elimination of fat mass. In fact, for these and other reasons, eating disorders such as Bulimia, Anorexia, Vomiting and Binge Eating Disorder mainly affect the female population, even if there are significant exceptions.

Eating disorders are described as pathologies characterized by alterations in eating habits and by excessive concern about one's image, in particular weight and body shapes.

Socio - Cultural Aspects

Social and cultural factors play a very important role in the genesis of food problems and pathologies. The great influence of the media and the continuous representations of models of physical perfection contribute significantly to the increase in cases of eating disorders with a significant and sometimes even devastating impact on adolescents and vulnerable subjects.

Therefore, guided by a distorted perception of their body and not by objective reality, these people obsessively seek perfection, which they identify in the unattainable reference models proposed by the mass media. The compulsive behavioral modalities typical of eating disorders are used to overcome negative states such as anxiety, inadequacy, low self-esteem and desire to please others.

The introduction of social media, has increased our exposure to images of retouched and artificial photos and consequent benchmarks far from reality. Although a direct link with the development of eating disorders is still to be demonstrated, it has been found that the emphasis placed by social media on the image is related to the development of greater anxiety towards the image itself, negatively affecting one's self-esteem.

Studies have shown that women and men who do not deal with the models conveyed by the mass media have a more positive perception of their image, as well as a better acceptance of their body shape.

In the face of globalized models of reference, the contradictory presence of mass media messages linked to food over-stimulation is associated. The result is a dissonant social communication which can in some predisposed subjects contribute to the onset and development of dysfunctional eating behaviors, with serious repercussions on health.

It is possible to do prevention of eating disorders in numerous ways. With the correct and appropriate knowledge on the topic of eating disorders, it is possible to convey more appropriate messages through a real social communication.

In this way, risk factors and the probability of spreading the disease can be transformed into preventive factors, making a significant contribution to tackling a problem of social relevance and promoting the adoption of healthy attitudes with respect to the perception of one's own body weight and shape.

Prevention Factors

With a view to the prevention of problems and disorders of eating behavior in adolescents, a fundamental role is played by educational action. The info about the nutritional properties of foods should be always considered, indicate the healthy foods to be taken and those that should be avoided. Since young age, at school, the competences for developing an individual capacity for critical evaluation should be transmitted. The educational purpose is to make consumers aware and immunized from the negative effects that many commercial messages can convey. In this way, we would become aware consumers rather than passive subjects who mechanically are exposed on business adverts on a daily basis.

At the basis of these disorders there are a series of factors that lead the person to delude himself that he can shift the control over food that one thinks he does not have over his life. Very often, one feels excessively worried about the judgment of others, influenced most of the time by the inability to establish meaningful social and personal relationships.

Factors Responsible for the Binge Eating Disorder

A sort of pendulum has often oscillated in the search for the factors responsible for eating disorders, going from organic to psychological and environmental factors. Today, the scientific community tends to propose multifactorial models for eating behavior disorders. It agrees that there is no single cause but a concomitance of factors that can differently interact with each other in favoring their appearance and perpetuation.

To have a correct idea about the development dynamics of the BED, a long series of factors that refer to a bio-psycho-social perspective must be kept in mind. This means that in the onset of an eating behavior disorder, factors that create a sort of predisposition or vulnerability come to interact. Genetic factors interact with cultural factors, on which other triggering factors act and precipitate the situation, which otherwise could remain latent. This in turn creates the conditions for the disease to perpetuate itself.

Predisposing Factors

Of the predisposing factors we will examine only some specific characteristics. Individual characteristics are some individual notes shared by people suffering from BED. These elements contribute to preparing a ground on which the disturbance of eating behavior can be grafted.

Registry Component

The first element is of a registry type. Teenagers are most vulnerable and most affected. Adolescence is an extremely delicate period of transition between childhood addiction and the autonomy of the adult phase. The eating disorder can arise from the inability to cope with these changes, the fear of maturity and all the requests and responsibilities it entails. In a certain sense, illness is a means, a way of staying or returning to children, in a protected situation both on the physical and on the emotional, cognitive and social levels.

Among the psychological factors, the idealization of thinness seems relevant. Skinny is good, fat is bad. This is the strong message that society sends. Girls know that men look at their bodies and are educated to be looked at. Having a body that respects the prevailing aesthetic canons becomes a sort of necessity for social relations.

Perfectionism

Generally there are personality traits characterized by perfectionism. These are ambitious people, with excellent results at school and in the activities they undertake, which show a commitment and tenacity often considered proof of great maturity and responsibility. This attitude of dedication and sacrifice almost always hides low self-esteem and profound personal insecurity, which expresses the fear of not being accepted by others for what you are.

The person thinks that he will be accepted only on condition that he gives his best without the slightest stretch mark. In people who get sick these traits are pushed to exasperation, any commitment that has nothing to do with the study or the activity on which it is invested is eliminated. The fear of disappointment and failure is great. The judgment of others is assessed as the only way to estimate one's worth. Many people are absolutely convinced that they are not as others would like them and they adapt to this idea by trying in every way to meet the expectations of others. They go on an obsessive search to trace the presence of a pathological perfectionism, due to an evaluation of themselves dependent by the achievement of certain very demanding and self-imposed personal standards. The judgment of others is considered the only way to estimate one's value.

Linked to perfectionism is a particular type of thought, called dichotomous thinking. Jumping from one extreme to another, there are no middle grounds, indeed half measures are not even considered. It is, therefore, a dichotomous personality, which moves between all or nothing, between moral contradictions, of thought and behavior. The obsessive lives on logic, in rationality and order, concepts that mix poorly with emotions.

In their relationship with others, they tend to lead, to make arrangements to be able to control better, and when they say something they actually give orders for being meticulously executed; only in this way do they satisfy their need for tranquility. They has no faith in anyone, delegating would be a risk, if they did, control and rules would fail.

Even emotions are subject to strict control, because if shown they are synonymous with weakness and vulnerability. They experience anger whenever they are unable to maintain control of their physical and interpersonal environment, however, they hardly express it directly, because they concentrate on what the others want, how to control addiction.

Before the disease becomes evident in many of these people traits of obsession, anxiety and depression are found. It is possible that these aspects are consequent to the state of malnutrition. The obsessive aspects, however, often seem to be pre-existing to the onset of the eating disorder.

Role of the family

The role of the family in the onset of an eating disorder has often been emphasized also inappropriately. The various theories that have dealt with this aspect have often referred to a disturbed relationship between mother and daughter. A particular configuration of family dynamics presents an overprotective, intrusive dominant mother and an absent father. In reality it is impossible to know whether a particular family climate is the cause rather than a consequence of the disturbance. It would be strange to imagine that in front of a daughter suffering from eating disorders, a parent does not become overprotective and that this does not cause a great increase in family tension.

What appears from the expanded observations of families with a BED-affected component is that there are a variety of different family situations and it is difficult to find common denominators. Today the idea that there is a typical family that favors the onset of anorexia is no longer accepted.

A separate consideration must be spent for those families in which there is a particular attention to the issues of physical appearance and nutrition. It is likely that a family atmosphere in which these aspects are emphasized could lead to the construction of a polarized self image on the external aspect. However, even in this case, there is no evidence that eating disorders occur more frequently in contexts of this type. Significant studies have shown that a high body dissatisfaction in parents favors a similar attitude.

The predisposing factors include, for example, pregnancy complications and perinatal damage, the presence of family members who suffer or have suffered from an eating disorder, have low self-esteem, interpersonal difficulties, body dissatisfaction and the use of low calorie diets. Risk factors are those factors that are capable of increasing the vulnerability to develop a particular disorder.

At the basis of these disorders there are a series of factors that lead the person to delude themselves that they can shift the control over food that one thinks they do not have over their life. Very often, one feels excessively worried about the judgment of others, influenced most of the time by the inability to establish meaningful social and personal relationships. Disorders of this kind can also occur following situations of severe stress or trauma.

Triggering Factors

The triggering factors are events that can determine the onset of the disorder in people who have a predisposition. They can be stressful or traumatic events such as bereavement, abuse, illness, family conflict, breaking an important relationship, changing school or city. In some cases it is not always easy to identify triggering events.

The fate of a person who presents a vulnerability to an eating disorder can be different depending on whether or not he or she encounters so-called triggering factors in his or her life which favor and determine the appearance of the actual disorder.

It is believed that undertaking a weight loss diet even in conditions of modest overweight, if there is a predisposition to the disorder, represents a crucial trigger. This obviously does not mean that all people who start a diet will experience an eating disorder. The combination of triggers seems to be the formula necessary for the manifestation of the disorder.

Sometimes the onset of weight gain is not associated with situations of body dissatisfaction but with adolescent problems, such as the impetuous changes that are observed during puberty development. The detachment from the family and the beginning or the end of an emotional relationship could be considered as other triggers. These are always events that tend to increase the difficulties encountered in terms of relationship skills and of one's autonomy and self-esteem, the change of residence, the loss of friends, the occurrence of physical or psychological harassment. At other times these are situations related to difficult and negative moments in life such as the death of a relative, a friend, an illness, a family crisis.

Usual Voluntary Actions

The current models for the search for triggers focus attention on three elements in particular. As for the first aspect, it must be remembered that the formation of a habit is the final result of an adaptive learning process.

Voluntary actions become habitual through reinforcement mechanisms. Overeating is the result of a learned habit. Environmental stimulus related to food, known as conditioned reinforcements, can sturdy increase the desire to eat even in the absence of food itself or in the absence of physiological needs related to hunger.

Through repeated pairing of a stimulus, a conditioned and unconditional stimulus with food, the learned stimulus becomes a salient incentive. It thus causes intense impulses to obtain the associated reward. It also acts as a conditioned reinforcement that contributes to maintaining the desire to seek food.

Habits can be considered compulsive when they persist despite devaluation. In compulsive nutrition, the inability to adapt eating behavior based on the motivational value of the result, may reflect a compulsive habit.

Compulsive behavior is hypothesized to reflect a maladaptive habit that previously constituted flexible and voluntary behavior.

Habits are formed through repeated action until the stimulus-response association interrupts the purpose of the behavior. For example, the search for a particular food represents a motivation to perform the action.

In some research it has been highlighted how compulsive behavior can be generated by a conflict or a stressful situation. In this case, this behavior tends to be characterized by its compulsive nature even when the triggering stimuli are absent. In other words, once this behavior has taken root, a sort of euphoric satisfaction is produced which produces addiction, comparable in all respects to substance dependence.

Maintenance Factors

The food restriction and the consequent decrease in weight, are all factors that over time promote depression, irritability and dissatisfaction with your body.

These factors, through a closed circuit mechanism, can induce a further food restriction, aimed at improving one's self-esteem.

It is very important to take these aspects into due consideration since, especially in the most serious and long-lasting situations, interventions should be aimed precisely at reducing these factors. In the impossibility of finding a precise cause to be removed, the most effective intervention is represented by the modification of those elements that keep the disorder alive.

Thought Aspects

Thought aspects are important initially. The ideas on weight and body shapes push the person to formulate a single thought regarding the physical aspect. This is followed by all those actions that can lead to the achievement of this goal. The intervention, in this case, must aim to question these defined dysfunctional assumptions. Often these ideas are reinforced from the outside, as it is not uncommon to find someone who compliments a normal weight who goes on a diet.

Over time, however, external reinforcement tends to decrease and the most important maintenance factor becomes the symptomatology determined by fasting. People who undergo a reduced diet, after a first phase characterized by euphoria and hyperactivity, develop a complex series of symptoms and signs that involve organic, behavioral and psychic aspects.

There are often important changes on the emotional level and depressive and irritability states emerge. Sometimes even more serious psychiatric manifestations can be found. A tendency to social isolation is often evident, amplified by the objective difficulties that the person suffering from BED in dating other people.

Friends, after a first moment, in which they encouraged the diet, become perplexed in the face of excessive weight gain and do not share their concerns about food. Furthermore, being together often involves convivial moments such as eating pizza or ice-cream. On these occasions, those suffering from BED only experience anxiety, embarrassment, desire for self-exclusion.

The onset of psychiatric symptomatology, anxiety, depression, irritability and the tendency to close in on themselves place the person in a condition in which any relationship is difficult, and even the acceptance of external help is problematic.

The person with an eating disorder has learned that controlling food is a powerful tool for controlling his anxieties and fear. Any attempt to reduce control can trigger a crisis of anxiety and depression.

After the initial phase, there is a decrease in the ability to concentrate, which often has to do with the need to increase any type of commitment. There is also a regression of the form of thought which becomes similar to that of the child, linked to the concrete data of everyday life and unable to elaborate hypotheses on the future. A situation occurs in which apathy, poor ability to concentrate are accompanied in a framework that tends to perpetuate the basic disorder.

As far as people with BED are concerned, the main factor of maintenance is the dominant thought of the binge which often becomes a diversion, a filler and an outlet that can appear more manageable against a crisis of anxiety and depression.

Over time, the person suffering from BED develops an inability to distinguish the different biological stimuli of hunger and satiety and to perceive to correctly manage anxiety, anger, loneliness and sadness.

They delude themselves that their bulimic eating behavior is a way to quell moments of anxiety and tension. Awareness of the resulting benefits is often minimal. The person who wants a cure is convinced that they want to change, but as the change looks forward they can realize that their determination is not so strong. The consequences are represented by feelings of guilt and personal disregard that can frustrate the drive to overcome the problem.

In these situations, a review of the motivation for treatment appears useful. In this sense it has always been said that bulimic behavior is experienced as negative and unpleasant.

The person suffering from BED would like to avoid binges but to assume a restrictive and controlled eating behavior, aimed at achieving that much desired body weight, but almost always too excessive, so he cannot maintain it.

The consequence would be above all in the fact that in the case of bulimia there is a more frequent request for help. Often the greatest willingness to care found in bulimia is only apparent. Beyond the declarations and also the real awareness of the person, the binge as abhorred is the means to quell anxiety. The moment when you give in to the temptation of food becomes a way to let go, to release tension, to give yourself forbidden food, to remove any negative thoughts. The binge is carefully planned, ensuring an adequate supply of food and eliminating any disturbing element.

Family Dynamics

Another factor of maintenance can be represented by family dynamics. The beginning of the problem can induce behaviors that, although perfectly understandable, unfortunately tend to perpetuate the disturbance.

The emergence of an overprotective attitude has the effect of reducing the autonomy of the subject. A situation of regression of the entire family is therefore created at a stage in which the parents had to deal completely with the feeding of the child.

If we consider that the engine of eating disorders is often represented by the fear of growing and becoming self-employed, it becomes evident how this situation can be more coherent with the maintenance of the disease. One modality that has proved particularly interesting for parents is that of self-help groups, where parents exchange experiences by providing mutual support. However a more careful reading of the situation can allow us to understand that these advantageous situations are nothing more than protective and defensive modalities that are assumed to face fear and difficulties.

5. CURE AND THERAPY

Proper Diagnostic Evaluation

For the treatment of eating disorders, it is important to contact specialist centers ideally expert with these problems. This will permit differential diagnosis to be made. The only way to understand if you suffer from a real eating disorder is to carry out all the necessary specialist psychological, psychiatric, internal and nutritional assessments. This is the only way to receive the correct information on the treatment to be followed.

Not all problems concerning eating behavior are real eating disorders.

A differential diagnosis allows us to understand if we are faced with other psychiatric diseases, such as depression or phobias, or with internal diseases such as celiac disease or endocrine problems.

The initial evaluation also has many other important objectives. First of all, it is the moment when a relationship of trust is established between the patient and the doctor. In the evaluation phase, all the information needed by the therapist is collected in order to understand which is the most appropriate path to follow.

The diagnostic evaluation generally lasts 2-4 visits made by a psychologist or psychiatrist and investigates the eating habits and attitudes regarding the patient's food and body. The social and family situation, school or work functioning and interpersonal relationships are assessed. In addition to the interview, the survey can also be conducted with interviews and questionnaires.

If the danger of medical complications is glimpsed, the diagnostic evaluation must be completed by an internal-nutritional examination. Finally, if the patient is under age, a visit for the parents is also indicated to complete the diagnostic picture. The point of view of the family members serves to establish an atmosphere of collaboration, as the family represents a point of trust even if the patient were to refuse or abandon therapy.

Care of the Binge Eating Disorder

An effective treatment of the Binge Eating Disorder disorder must take into consideration the medical-internal part, the nutritional part and the more strictly psychological part.

The main problem is therefore the close connection between emotion and food. Food becomes a tool to anesthetize negative emotions. At the same time, however, the Binge conducts lead to feelings of guilt and unease. This creates a vicious circle harmful to the patient's physical and mental health.

This is a psychological and emotional disorder that encloses a very painful personal situation.

For most people with BED, the awareness of having a problem is low and the fear of facing a change is very strong. Eating without control, extreme diets, can be seen by the person suffering from BED not so much as a disturbance, but rather as a solution to their problems. This disturbance is so pervasive that it leads to the illusion of being able to keep other life problems away. In fact, many problems are caused by the eating disorder itself.

This is the reason why many people with eating disorders, especially in the early stages of the disease, do not ask for help or even refuse a therapeutic approach. Many epidemiological studies have found that people with BED ask for therapeutic help. In any case, the therapeutic contact allows in these cases to open a dialogue and to monitor any complications, both medical and psychological.

If a person with an eating disorder is not yet able to undertake a real treatment, a motivational path is usually started. That is, a psychological path that aims to bring the person to desire change and healing.

Being motivated to change means feeling an unease that gives the awareness of getting involved and the courage to ask for help. A collaboration between different professional figures who deal in an integrated way with these disorders that can be psychiatric with important psychopathological manifestations.

The most effective approach for the treatment of eating disorders is the multidisciplinary and integrated one.

How to Choose the Treatment

When a person with eating disorders arrives in a specialized facility, a correct and careful diagnostic evaluation with a multidisciplinary and integrated approach for more or less intensive treatment is essential.

It is always a good rule to start, except for specific contraindications, from the less intensive treatment, i.e. outpatient treatment, because it interferes less with the social life of the person. Only in cases where outpatient treatment has not worked will more intensive treatment be used, such as semi-residential day-hospital treatment.

The choice to carry out a therapeutic program in hospitalization regime is made when there are medical complications, such as a very high frequency of bulimic crises, improper use of drugs, multi-impulsivity, self-aggressive behavior, high suicidal risk and failure to previous treatments.

The most suitable treatment for the person must be chosen together with a trusted therapist after a thorough diagnostic evaluation. The factors to be considered are the type of disorder, the physical situation, the presence of complications, the duration of the disease, the age, the person's expectations, previous therapeutic experiences and the characteristics of the patient's personalities.

Nutritional Treatment

The performance of the nutritional program will ensure that you are able to prevent loss of control over your diet or sudden weight gains. This point is very important and must be shared with patients who obviously have many fears and concerns in facing food and changing habits.

The aim of nutritional rehabilitation is to gradually restore correct nutrition by inserting the foods considered taboo in a guided and gradual way and contrasting the trend towards dietary restriction. Therefore, both the quantity of food and the quality problems are tackled, including those considered fattening and therefore phobic. The path must be carefully guided taking into account the patient's fears and duration of illness. Discomfort may initially arise due to digestive difficulties resulting from a prolonged restriction.

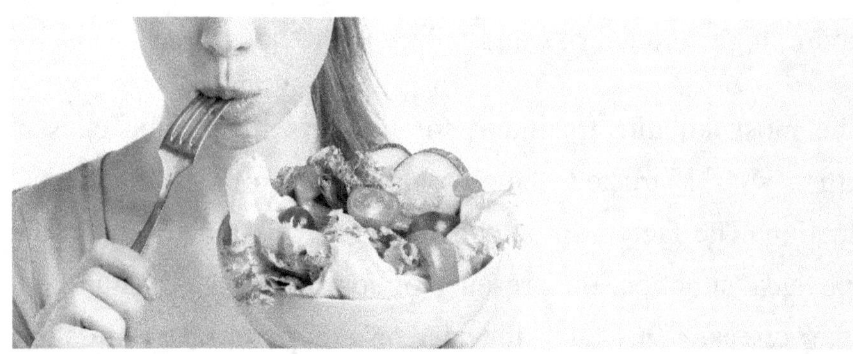

The food program is divided into 3 main meals plus 1 or 2 snacks. In outpatient treatment, the division of meals throughout the day, the portions of the courses and the type of food to be included are agreed with the therapist, tested at home, verified and discussed in the next meeting.

The Pharmacological Treatment

Pharmacological treatments are based on antidepressants, serotonergic, that is, serotonin reuptake inhibitors such as citalopram or paroxetine. They work correctly, but they have the defect that after a few months the results go down. Having reached this last stage, the subject is able to limit binge eating. Obviously, if in the meantime the personality or the experience evolves positively, all the causes at the origin of the depression will also be removed, making the compensation mechanism underlying the Binge Eating Disorder useless.

The use of drugs is linked to the observation that other psychopathologies are often associated with these disorders, such as depressive and obsessive-compulsive disorders. For this reason, the most frequently used drugs are antidepressant drugs with mainly serotonergic action. The pharmacological treatment of eating disorders should never be considered as the main treatment, but always as a supportive treatment for psychotherapeutic or psychoeducational work.

In bulimia nervosa, antidepressant therapy has shown specific efficacy in reducing bulimic symptoms and in reducing associated psychic symptoms, such as depression, obsessive symptoms and impulsivity. The long-term efficacy of antidepressant therapy remains poorly understood and the clinical impression is that even in bulimia nervosa antidepressant treatment can only be effective in association with psychotherapeutic treatments. The use of mood stabilizing drugs, associated with antidepressant therapy, can be useful in the treatment of anorexia nervosa and bulimia nervosa when they are associated with multi-impulsive characteristics.

Psychological Treatment

Psychological treatments are based on the control of food intake, on the variation of eating habits, up to a real food consciousness.

The psychological treatment proposed for eating disorders considers the presence of incorrect or distorted knowledge about food and one's body as the main responsible for pathological attitudes and eating behaviors. Behaviors such as food restriction, avoidance and weight and body control behaviors are in turn factors for maintaining distorted cognitions. In psychological therapy, therefore, both incorrect eating behaviors and related cognitive style are addressed.

The Cognitive-Behavioral Model

TCB model essentially consists of three main phases. In the first phase, the patient is given information on the disorder, the aim is to reduce binge eating and regularize the frequency and composition of meals with alternative activities to bulimic crises.

In the second phase, the goal is to improve the quality and quantity of nutrition, to face the idea of a diet, to recognize risky situations and to practice problem solving exercises.

In the third phase, the results obtained are consolidated and the topic of relapse prevention is addressed. A very useful technique is the use of the food diary, in which the mode and quantity of nutrition, the emotions and beliefs related to food are recorded by the patient. Through this self-monitoring, patients learn to recognize and avoid risky situations and behaviors, obviously after having analyzed everything with the therapist.

In reality, the TCB uses a global approach called transdiagnostic. In a first phase of the treatment, it focuses on managing the acute phase of the eating disorder and subsequently the therapy plans to address all the problems associated with the eating disorder, family difficulties, relationships and the development of a fragile self-esteem.

Cognitive Behavioral Therapy can be individual or group. The group approach has been successfully used for bulimia nervosa and in uncontrolled feeding disorder. Review and meta-analysis studies have highlighted the effectiveness of these treatments on the evolution of symptoms and on the improvement of the psychopathological picture. The sense of shame, of secrecy that characterizes bulimic crises, interpersonal difficulties, isolation and low self-esteem lead the subject to increase feelings of guilt and a sense of inadequacy. The group can become a place of reflection, comparison and transformation.

Interpersonal Psychotherapy

Developed by Klerman in 1994 for the treatment of depression, it has been extended to the treatment of bulimia nervosa and BED. This addresses the difficulties of interpersonal relationships designed at the basis of eating disorders.

Interpersonal psychotherapy involves a first phase in which the focus of the treatment is identified. A thematic area is addressed by choosing from 4 categories, difficulties in forging and maintaining significant ties, conflicts with relatives and friends, difficulties in role changes and unprocessed bereavements.

In the next phase the patient takes on a more active role and is invited to talk about his current difficulties and to experiment with new relationship models to relate them to the focus of the problem that has been previously identified to prepare the patient for the problems they will face in the future.

Psychoanalytic Psychotherapy

Psychoanalysis assumes that the symptoms are the expression of unconscious conflicts. Psychoanalytic psychotherapy acts mainly on what are considered to be the predisposing factors for dietary pathology. Its goal is to allow the maintenance of the results achieved through the analysis and resolution of internal conflicts and interpersonal problems. Through introspection, the patient discovers and analyzes these conflicts.

The psychoanalytic approach is useful if the physical and psychic consequences of the symptoms are not such as to prevent psychological work. It is therefore advisable to undertake this type of therapy only once the weight has been recovered or the frequency of bulimic crises has improved in order to address the underlying psychological problems.

Food Psychoeducation

Psychoeducation is an educational technique that aims to raise awareness of the mechanisms by which a particular disorder has arisen, is maintained and can be cured. It takes into account patients' rights to be fully informed and improves adherence to treatments because it involves the patient in the therapeutic choices.

As for eating disorders, very often wrong and distorted information and beliefs circulate about the caloric content of food. Psychoeducational techniques consist in providing correct information on the properties of nutrients, on the metabolic functioning, on the biological effects of restrictive diets, on the reasons of amenorrhea, on the relationship between weight loss and physical and psychological symptoms.

In some initial and non-serious cases, psychoeducation, together with some nutritional advice, can in itself lead to a remission of the symptoms. The absence of at least one regular meal a day or the use of compensatory methods shows the need for more specific help. Isolation and poor social support are other factors that make the success of a purely psychoeducational intervention difficult. In general, therefore, psychoeducation can be considered a very useful therapeutic technique, but which must be associated with other therapeutic interventions.

Family Therapy

Family therapy is an important part of treatment, as it involves and works with families. The goal of family therapy is to promote change, with sessions supervised by a family therapist.

Family therapy must be considered when a malfunction is observed within a family. It helps to highlight problems concerning the general ability of the family to respond to emotions under stress. This form of therapy can be useful to eliminate those potentially lethal situations for the BED, of which the family very often contributes to the cause despite being unaware of it.

An advanced version of this therapy is called the Maudsley Method. This family-based treatment focuses on involving parents as an active role in the recovery process of the child from eating disorders. This would include parental guidance in helping their child eat balanced and healthy meals and prevent deviant behavior.

Several studies suggest the usefulness of treatments aimed at family members with the aim of improving knowledge related to the disease and its treatment and to decrease the family burden and excessive emotional involvement.

Family therapies can help parents better understand the pathological aspects of their child's behavior and can be helpful in interrupting the vicious circle of the disease.

The goal of family therapies is not to search for the causes of the disease but to have possible co-therapists within the family, to better contribute to the success of the treatment. Often these are apparently simple tasks, such as easing the tension at mealtimes, but which require good control so that it is better to behave in one way rather than another. This is the psychoeducational approach that involves providing information on eating disorders and their treatments in order to improve collaboration in treatment.

Cognitive Rehabilitation Therapy

Cognitive rehabilitation therapy is a treatment that is born for people resistant to treatments. It is an intervention that can be used both as a pre-treatment program and as an additional module to cognitive-behavioral psychotherapies.

It is an intervention that consists of mental exercises aimed at improving cognitive strategies. The assumptions on which the program is based are constituted by the idea that the brain and the process of information are not given once and for all, but that they are able to change throughout life if subjected to specific training.

The purpose of the treatment is to help the patient acquire a series of strategies that facilitate the acquisition of greater thinking flexibility. The patient will be put in a position to adopt a more global style of thinking, against the tendency towards excessive attention to detail.

It is a slightly different approach from the classic psychotherapeutic interventions. It mainly addresses how the patient thinks and not the content of thought. No emphasis is placed on the food symptoms manifested by the person, but attention is paid to the thought processes through the use of simple and specific cognitive exercises different and far from nutrition and weight. This generally reduces the patient's resistance by improving adherence to therapy (compliance). It consists of mental exercises aimed at improving cognitive strategies, thinking skills and the acquisition of information through practice, to promote a reflection on thinking styles. It helps explore new thinking strategies in everyday life.

Self-help Group

By reading and using self-help manuals on the market on eating disorders, the patient tries to solve their problem on their own.

A number of people suffering from eating disorders gather in groups according to the rules of anonymous alcoholics to fight the eating disorder, usually the BED more rarely than the bulimia nervosa.

Reading and using self-help manuals are combined with the support of a professional. The patient can also be guided in this form of therapy by the general practitioner, a dietician or a social worker. There are studies that have proven the effectiveness of pure and guided self-help in patients with non-serious forms of eating disorder and there are several manuals.

CONCLUSION

This book is mainly aimed at subjects affected by Binge Eating Disorder, to stimulate them to adopt more balanced lifestyles aimed at psychophysical well-being. At the same time, we wanted to give indications to many people on how to avoid health risks deriving from incorrect information on eating disorders.

Eating disorders are psychiatric conditions that use the body as a means of expressing frustrations. For this reason, it is extremely important to implement a diagnostic approach that takes into consideration the organic, psychological and social endocrine components.

Patients who are affected by these disorders often have very serious organic complications. Generally, it is the symptoms that lead the patient, driven by family members, to a first contact with the doctor. In most cases these subjects diminish the entire symptomatological spectrum.

The treatment of patients with these pathologies varies based on the type of disorder and the level of impairment of the patient's health. The integration of multiple specialists in the therapeutic planning and management of these patients remains the most suitable form of intervention. With these patients, the first thing to do is to establish a very close exchange of trust before starting a therapeutic relationship.

The therapist will conduct an accurate and detailed history of the subject's history to understand the individual factors related to the development of the disorder. The clinical experiences reported by the therapists come to the conclusion that the patients' experiences, their traumas are considered risk factors predisposing to the development of psychiatric and food disorders. Therapy will be characterized by a remarkable flexibility of a program, which gradually adapts to the intellectual abilities and experiences passed by the various patients.

In fact, the main objective of this work concerns the origin and evolutionary path of BED. The most effective contrast to this disorder is given by the possibility of resorting to a global therapeutic program, which focuses on both memories and situations present, which cause emotional distress.

In patients with eating disorders, there is a strong tendency to isolate and avoid contact with others. The traumatic experience can upset the existence of an individual causing negative feelings of distrust towards themselves and towards others and altering emotional patterns.

Appropriate therapies help the patient to construct information constructively and to experience what he feels within himself. Guilt and shame are progressively transformed into adequate responsibility of an adult being, who make their choices confidently. The solution of the disorder is achieved through the stimulation of the patient's innate self-healing processes. The information processing mechanism is physiologically designed to solve psychological disorders in the same way that the rest of the body is equipped to heal a physical injury.

When the patient has worked out his frustrations, he will also be able to recall the positive events that have occurred, which allow him to redefine himself as a person of positive abilities, with a past and a future. The patient's evaluation of himself changes, thanks to the internal emotion processing system that is stimulated, so that the healthy nucleus that is already present can emerge.

Cognitive behavioral therapy is today the most effective treatment for the treatment of these disorders. It regulates the eating style through psycho educational encounters, which make it possible to know useful information to deal with and resolve the disorder and the prevention of possible relapses.

Patients with eating disorders become aware of their abilities and leave the sense of emptiness to increase their self-control. Interpersonal psychotherapy allows the reworking of past and present events that cause disturbance, teach patients to value the past, to plan the future and manage stress without resorting to binge eating.

Through these programs, people suffering from Binge Eating Disorder can learn to manage their emotions and thoughts and can develop a healthy relationship with food.